Butter Coffee Weight Loss Protocol

Harness the Power of Butter Coffee & MCT Oil for Fat Loss

By Greg Cook

Table of Contents

Copyright

contained within is the solitary and utter responsibility of the recipient reader.

Under no circumstances will any legal responsibility or blame be held against the publisher for any reparation, damages, or monetary loss due to the information herein, either directly or indirectly. Respective authors own all copyrights not held by the publisher.

The information herein is offered for informational purposes solely, and is universal as so. The presentation of the information is without contract or any type of guarantee assurance.

The trademarks that are used are without any consent, and the publication of the trademark is without permission or backing by the trademark owner. All trademarks and brands within this book are for clarifying purposes only and are the owned by the owners themselves, not affiliated with this document.

Introduction

Weight affects health. People who have excess weight are more prone to develop certain diseases such as diabetes, heart problems, cancer s and stroke. Weight loss is most often a very difficult goal to achieve. One great, easy yet effective way to lose weight is by following the Butter Coffee Weight Loss Protocol.

This weight loss regimen incorporates all the health benefits of coffee, butter and MCT oil to lose weight and achieve a healthier body. The main thing about this protocol is to drink butter coffee daily. Yes, butter in coffee.

Find out more about this unique, revolutionary and definitely out-of-the-box method to get the healthier and fitter body you deserve.

Chapter 1: What Is Butter Coffee?

Butter coffee is a term used for brewed coffee that is blended with butter or MCT (medium chain triglycerides) oil. The practice was introduced by Dave Asprey. He reportedly felt rejuvenated when he was served yak butter tea by locals after he hiked in Tibet at 18,000 feet in a minus 10-degree weather.

Benefits of Butter Coffee

Supporters of butter coffee report several benefits gained from daily intake of this one-of-a-kind beverage, such as the following:

Fat Loss

The biggest and most popular benefit from butter coffee is fat loss. Some experts believe that MCT in butter helps in losing adipose or fatty tissues in the body.

More Energy

Those who take butter coffee report having more energy to perform daily functions. This is because of the MCT added, which many studies have found to be a good quick source of energy. MCTs are oxidized by the body rapidly, which leads to the increase in the energy expenditure. It is also absorbed differently by the body compared to other forms of fats, such as the LCFA or long chain fatty acids.

How Butter Coffee Works

According to the proponent, Dave Asprey, each ingredient plays important roles in achieving the many benefits.

Coffee

There are many conflicting studies about the health benefits of coffee. The caffeine content in ordinary coffee gives a good boost, which is why lots of people take it for breakfast.

It helps to jumpstart the day with increased energy, better concentration and improved focus. However, most coffee in the market contains toxins. The toxins can come anywhere from the many processes that the coffee beans pass through. It may come from pesticides, insecticides and chemical fertilizers used during the growing of the coffee plant. Or, from the preservatives and other chemicals during the harvest, transport, roasting, and manufacturing processes that the coffee beans may undergo. Also, plain coffee would provide the desired buzz for a limited time. On the average, the boost would only last for 2 hours. Afterwards, one would generally feel the craving, crash and tiredness. Anyone used to having coffee for breakfast would be familiar with the 10:30 AM crash. By adding the other ingredients, i.e., MCT oil and butter, these won't likely happen.

MCT

Medium chain triglycerides used in butter coffee comes from a special blend of palm oil and coconut oil. MCT behaves more like carbohydrates than oil in the body. It is quickly metabolized and turned into readily usable energy. This is also responsible for the weight loss that a lot of practitioners report to achieve.

Butter

Blending butter into coffee and MCT oil helps to address cravings. When the energy crashes as the effect of caffeine wanes, cravings start and maybe difficult to control. Micronutrients in butter help to supply energy and nutrition to the brain, turning off the cravings.

Also, there are some compounds in butter that can decrease inflammation that may be present in the brain. The type of butter is also important. Ordinary butter is often full of inflammatory compounds that can come from lots of sources. Hormones and antibiotics given to most cows to improve growth and milk production can trigger inflammation in the body. Butter used in butter coffee should come from the milk of grass-fed cows, which were not treated with hormones and antibiotics.

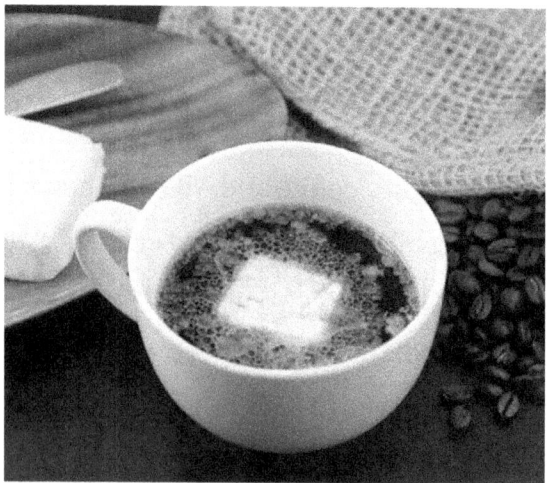

Image: blog.fitbit.com

Chapter 2: Pros and Cons

There are so many debates going on about the effectiveness of butter coffee, not only in terms of weight loss but also of its effects on health. Here are some of the pros and cons that have surfaced regarding this unique and rather odd beverage.

PROS

According to those who support the Butter Coffee Weight Loss Protocol, butter and MCT oil are the main factors that produce the health benefits. In order to get the most benefits, only grass-fed butter is used. Otherwise, butter coffee would only pack in a huge amount of calories without any substantial benefit on health.

Fats

Omega-3 and Omega-6 in grass-fed butter

The fats in grass-fed butter are the healthy kind. It is believed to help in regulating the cholesterol levels in the body.

It does not lead to higher cholesterol levels, like most people are led to believe. In fact, grass-fed butter contains the best ratio of omega-3 and omega-6 fatty acids. This ratio is very important when consuming omega-6 and omega-3. An average Western diet has too much omega-6 and too little of omega-3. Most people think that eating lots of omega-3 and/or omega-6 is enough to create a healthy lipid profile in the body. This isn't the whole picture. Too much of either is bad for the health. High intake of omega-6 leads to increased inflammatory conditions in the body. High omega-3 intake inhibits inflammation, which puts the body more prone to injuries and tissues damage. Inflammation is not always bad. It has protective effects in the body, as long as it is controlled and localized. One should maintain a good balance of intake of these 2 fatty acids in order to get the health benefits. The recommended ratio of omega-6 to omega-3 in the daily intake is at 1:1 to 5:1. Higher ratios have been found to increase the risk for cancers, cardiovascular disease and autoimmune disorders.

Aside from improving inflammatory conditions, the fats in grass-fed butter are also special. These are biologically active. This means that the body has other uses for it besides as energy sources. These fats play important roles in different bodily processes such as blood clotting.

Of the commonly used oils and fats in food and food preparation, coconut oil and butterfat rank among the lowest in polyunsaturated fatty acids.

Here is a comparison:

- Sunflower oil – contains 71% omega-6, 1% omega-3
- Peanut oil – contains 33% omega-6 and only minute amounts of omega-3
- Canola oil – contains 21% polyunsaturated fat (omega-6) in the

form of linoleic acid, 11% omega-3 (in the form of alpha-linolenic acid)

- Flaxseed oil – contains 18% omega-6 fatty acid, 57% omega-3
- Palm oil – 10% omega-6
- Lard – contains 9% omega-6 and 1% omega-3
- Olive oil – 9% omega-6 and 1% omega-3
- Butterfat – contains 3% omega-6 and 1% omega-3
- Coconut oil – contains 2% omega-6

In fact, the American Heart Association lists raw, unprocessed butter from grass-fed cows as among the healthy sources of fats, along with coconut oil.

Other types of fats present in grass-fed butter

There are still other types of fats found in grass-fed butter that has health benefits. Some of them are used in building cell membranes, which is necessary in repair and replacement of damaged tissues, hormone synthesis and for growth. One special kind of fat found in butter is butyrate, a short chain fatty acid. This fat was previously thought to be bad for the health. However, newer studies found that butyrate is linked to the prevention of degenerative diseases that affect the nervous system, such as Alzheimer's and Parkinson's. This short chain fatty acid also increases the body's energy expenditure and reduces inflammation. These characteristics help in further preventing the development of heart diseases.

Coconut oil

Coconut oil is added as an alternative to pure MCT oil. This does not contain significant amounts of omega-3 or omega-6, but is rich in medium chain fatty acids (MCFAs). It contains beneficial types of fats that can help boost the body's immune system, metabolism, thyroid function and skin health.

MCT

MCT is known for its health boosting, metabolic-raising and muscle building effects. In fact, lots of muscle builders and athletes are turning to MCT oil for quick energy boosts as well as aid in promoting endurance and muscle building. Medium chain fatty acids behave very differently than other types of fats. It is metabolized by the body much like carbohydrates, but without the blood sugar raising and insulin-stimulating effects. MCT does not go through the long process of digestion.

It is quickly converted by the body into readily usable energy, making it

perfect as a quick energy source. It also does not affect the cholesterol and lipid profile of the body like long chain triglycerides do.

Nutrients

Aside from the healthy kinds of fats found in grass-fed butter, there Rae also other nutrients that can be obtained from it.

Better cognitive function

Caffeine boosts the mind's functioning. However, the effect lasts only for a short while. By adding butter and MCT oil, the effect of caffeine is prolonged. Also, the compounds found in grass-fed butter and MCT oil enhances the brains functioning, making one more focused with better cognitive function. Also, the mood enhancing effects of the fats in butter helps in reducing stress. A relaxed mind and body work well together, achieving more and becoming more productive.

Butter coffee also helps the body in fat burning to produce ketones. These ketones are used by the body as energy to fuel different functions and processes. This is a better energy source for the brain than glucose from carbohydrates.

Weight loss

Aside from the beneficial effects of the different types of fats in butter and coconut oil in butter coffee, this concoction can also help in losing weight.

The fats help the body feel full and satiated longer, reducing the hunger. Grass-fed butter also contains the compounds CLA or conjugated linoleic acid. Studies have found that this compound can help in reducing the body fat mass. Overweight individuals can get the most benefit from CLA. Taking butter coffee in the morning packs in a lot of healthy calories.

The energy from butter and the boost from coffee work together to stimulate fat burning that lasts for most of the day.

A cup of butter coffee in the morning, according to practitioners can replace an entire meal. The energy from the fats is a better energy source that leads to higher performance compared to glucose. Glucose in the blood is quickly removed from the blood as the cells use it for fuel or stored due to the presence of insulin. Once glucose enters the blood, insulin is quickly activated to get as much of it stored inside the cells. Hence, the body has to be quick to get some of it used as energy before everything is stored up, leaving an energy deficit. This leads to the crash and the craving. The body has to obtain much needed energy in order to perform and carry out its many homeostatic processes. In response to the deficit, the body prompts itself to seek for quick sources energy, leading to the cravings. Once a person eats, the process starts all over again. With butter and MCT oil, the body has a steady supply of energy.

These fat sources are slowly digested, releasing slow but steady stream of energy that body can have access to at any time. And because fats do not raise the blood sugar levels and trigger insulin release, these fats do not get to be stored as quickly as glucose. The body no longer needs to feel the need to feed because it still has a readily available supply of energy for all its needs.

CONS

There are some disadvantages in taking butter coffee, too. These include the following:

Taking low-nutrient food

Butter coffee is packed with energy that a person needs to get through most of the morning. A person does not feel hungry in the middle of the day, which reduces snacking. The feeling of fullness can often extend over to lunch hour, which leads to eating less amount of food. In short, a person taking butter coffee to start the day feels less hungry throughout the day.

For most people, a cup of butter coffee in the morning can replace a good breakfast meal. Butter coffee is not a complete meal, however. It has essentially just a few vitamins and antioxidants (from butter and coffee). A person has to take supplements in order to get the complete nutrients needed to ensure a healthy body.

Taste

Most people who tried butter coffee report that their coffee tastes better, creamier because of the added grass-fed butter. A few report it tasting awful. People have different tastes preferences and there is no getting around this fact. Also, some people do not like the greasy feel on their lips after they sip their coffee. However, the taste may be improved by placing coffee, butter and MCT oil in a powerful blender. The large fat droplets will be broke into tiny ones, which will reduce the oiliness of the beverage.

Chapter 3: Weight Loss Protocol

The goal of the Butter Coffee Weight Loss Protocol is to stimulate the body to metabolize fats and lose as much as possible. Before starting this weight loss protocol, consult a doctor. Have a complete checkup and laboratory tests. These will serve as baseline data to base the improvements or progress after following the diet protocol. The checkup will also determine if there are possible contraindications or if any adjustments may be needed.

So, to achieve weight loss safely and effectively using the Butter Coffee Weight Loss Protocol, follow these easy steps:

Step 1: Drink Butter Coffee

Mix together high quality (upgraded) coffee, MCT oil and grass-fed butter. Start with a small amount of MCT in the recipe.

Too much too soon can cause a few gastrointestinal upset such as cramps and diarrhea. Allow the body some time to adjust to the oils, especially if this is the first time to add coconut or MCT oils to the daily meals.

Drink as much butter coffee in the morning, depending on caffeine tolerance. It is recommended, though, to limit the first week to a cup in the morning. This would be about 500mL or less of butter coffee. Increase the intake as the body- and the palate- has adjusted to this concoction. Butter coffee can be taken in the afternoon, too, around 2PM. This can be done if feeling hungry or tired in the afternoon- for a quick energy and mental boost, as well as fat burning. How much and how often butter coffee is consumed is subject to caffeine tolerance. However, it is highly recommended to avoid drinking butter coffee after 2 PM because it may interrupt with nighttime sleep. Also, do not eat anything during the day.

If feeling hungry but not too keen on having another cup of coffee, drink water or tea instead. Or eat butter sprinkled with a small amount of salt for improved taste.

Step 2: Choosing the right food and exercise

Part of the Butter Coffee Weight Loss Protocol is choosing what other food to eat. During the 5 to 6days of the 1st week into the diet protocol, do not eat any carbohydrate- or protein-containing foods. Have a food day after this period. Keep well hydrated, too. This is very important in order to flush out toxins and prevent dehydration. Water also helps in further boosting metabolism and energy levels.

Even with the dietary restrictions, most people report feeling better, less hungry, better focus and mental alertness, as well as feeling more energetic.

This is because the fast in butter coffee provides all the body's energy needs to get through all of the day's activities. Some people even feel super charged. This may come from the boosting effect of caffeine as well as the ketones. Again, ketones are energy forms generated from fat metabolism. However, experts agree that it is not a good idea to use the energy from ketones to get some heavy exercise. While ketones do make one feel amped, it won't help in achieving exercise goals. It can cause a few difficulties when it comes to strength training and muscle-building. Ketones can make it difficult to achieve muscle mass through exercise. A short, light to medium type of workout once a week is ideal, but nothing heavy or too strenuous.

Also, some people may need to take digestive aids to help in digesting and emulsifying the fats in coffee.

A capsule of Betaine HCl can help. A person who isn't used to this much fat in the diet may have a few unwanted side effects such as bloating, cramping and diarrhea.

Step 3: Take Supplements

Because 5 to 6 days of pure fat intake, the body is missing out on other important nutrients. Take supplements to provide for the body's nutrient needs. Here are some of the most important supplements to take during this period:

Vitamin D – Target levels is at 70 to 90. Take 1000 IU per 25 pounds of the body's weight. For example, for a person weighing 150 pounds, take daily vitamin supplements at 6000 IU.

Magnesium and Potassium – To be taken at night. Take 500 mg of magnesium and 200 mg of potassium supplements.

Krill oil - take 1 capsule of krill oil a day, together with butter coffee.

Vitamin K2 – Take 2000 mcg a day, about 1 capsule.

Unbuffered Vitamin C – take about 1 to 2 grams every 8 hours

Glutathione – This is important to support liver function. Take 1 teaspoon twice per day.

BCAA (Branched Chain Amino Acids) – this will supply the protein needs for the day. Take 5 grams twice each day.

Coconut charcoal – This helps in binding with toxins in the body and aids in flushing it all out. Take 2 o 10 capsules, about twice or thrice per day.

During the 1st week into the Butter Coffee Weight Loss Protocol, a few discomforts may arise. The 1st 3 days would be when the most discomforts would be felt.

Headaches may develop, as well as symptoms resembling flu (e.g., muscle aches, fatigue, etc). These discomforts are due to the adjustments that the body makes because of the changes. These will eventually pass without much incident after a couple of days. Never take any medication during this time, even for the headaches. Medications at this point can harm the liver. These will also interfere with the action of glutathione. Drink lots of water. Most often, headaches are due to dehydration.

About 8 pounds will be rapidly lost during the first week. This is mainly due to the loss of glycogen stores and water. Then, a plateau will occur over the next few days. This means no weight loss or gain. This does not mean that the diet is no longer working. This is just an indication that the body is finding its balance based on the new diet plan. After the plateau, weight loss will happen again.

This time, weight is lost in chunks, and then another plateau, followed by as much as 3 to 5 pounds lost in 1 day.

At anytime that a person feels unwell during the weight loss protocol, stop the diet and consult with a doctor. Though safe, some people may need to adjust some parts of the diet to match individual health conditions and needs.

Step 4: Re-feed

After 5 to 6 days of purely subsisting on fat, time to re-feed. This will keep the body's hormonal levels at fat-burning levels. Prolonged deprivation of carbohydrates and proteins can place the body in defensive mode. That is, it will severely inhibit fat loss ad increase fat storage. Also, prolonged low protein intake may cause the body to digest protein stores, such as those in the muscles, which can lead to muscle loss.

Re-feed day is not cheat day. That is, this day does not mean uncontrollable eating of anything and everything. Watch the food choices on this day. Still avoid high sugar foods and junk foods, which are always unhealthy and should be completely removed from the diet. Eating these kinds of foods can throw all the past few days of hard work down the drain. Eat starchy tubers, for starters, such as sweet potatoes. Eat also large amounts of healthy proteins such as meat from grass-fed animals, wild seafood (i.e., wild salmon, tuna, herring, etc) and pastured eggs.

Some people would gain 1-2 pounds after the re-feed day. This is no cause for alarm. This is more likely from retained water because of the carbohydrates. All these will be lost and more once the 5 to6 days of butter coffee-only days are resumed.

Step 5: Retest

Consult the doctor again and take the same laboratory tests taken at the start of the protocol. This will track progress. Most likely, the HDL levels will be increased, as more toxins in the body are being metabolized.

Also, body fat percentage would drop, too. Most people report a 10 to 14% drop in body fat while on this weight loss protocol.

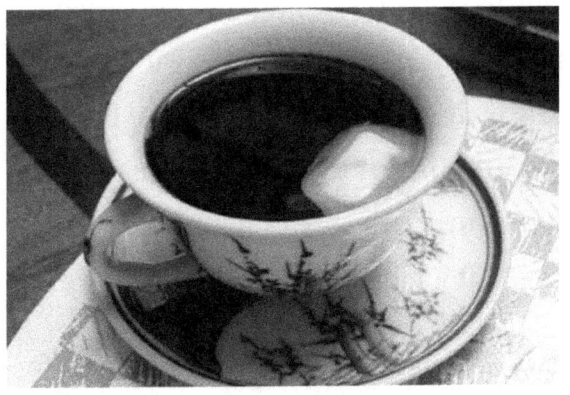

Image: http://www.whydontyoutrythis.com

Higher mTOR

mTOR means mammalian target of rapamycin. This is a major mechanism in the body that increases the rate of protein synthesis in the muscles. Everyone, particularly people who have weight issues, should get excited about higher mTOR. This mechanism helps in building more muscle mass, which can reduce fat storage (i.e., improve fat burning and lose weight). The mechanism starts by raising the rate by which the muscle cells use energy. This will temporarily inhibit the body's muscle building system. After the brief cessation, muscle building returns at a higher pace. This will lead to gaining more muscle mass as one eats.

This means that the energy from food is used for gaining muscles instead of getting converted into fat and stored, which leads to weight gain.

There are basically 3 major ways of increasing

mTOR. These include intermittent fasting, coffee and exercise. Resveratrol (in grapes and grape wine), turmeric, green tea and chocolate are also known to increase mTOR, but on a much lesser scale. Butter Coffee Weight Loss Protocol utilizes all of the 3 major mTOR boosters. Intermittent fasting is actually the 5 to6 days of pure butter coffee intake. Exercise is also part of the diet protocol, which should be light to moderate only. Most importantly, coffee. All these 3 work together to boost muscle building, leading to leaner, healthier and fitter body.

Ketosis

Ketosis is a process by which the body burns or converts fats into energy forms called ketones. This simply means fat burning to provide energy for the body to use, especially the brain. This is stimulated by removing carbohydrates from the diet, which prompts the body to rely on fats for energy. Often, ketosis stops once a person eats carbohydrates again, which is on re-feed day. By adding MCT oil in butter coffee, ketosis continues even while eating small amounts of carbohydrates. Also, the presence of MCT oil helps the body to enter ketosis much sooner than usual. This oil helps to promote faster and prolonged ketosis compared to just grass-fed butter and coffee.

Feel better

Regular fasting to lose weight can leave a person cranky, sluggish, preoccupied with hunger, unable to focus, weak, and tired most of the time. This can spell serious trouble for people who have to go to school or work. Reduced productivity is not a good trade-off to shed a few pounds. With the Butter Coffee Weight Loss Protocol these unwanted side effects are eliminated. One can still work and function at normal levels even while on fasting mode. The fats in MCT and butter provide all the needed energy. And because the body uses ketones, mood is improved as well as cognitive function. The steady supply of energy from fats and ketones also helps the body feel more energized and feel better even while on a fast.

Higher metabolic rates

Other types of weight loss diets do not affect the metabolic rates. Higher metabolic rates are needed in order to sustain weight loss. Coffee is known to boost metabolism by as much as 20%.

Therefore, the combination of coffee, MCT oil and grass-fed butter is a potent mix to boost health and achieve safe and effective, as well as sustainable weight loss.

Chapter 4: How to Make Butter Coffee

There are lots of variations on how butter coffee is made. Some add a few herbs and spices such as cinnamon to make it more palatable and flavorful.

The basic recipe is as follows:

Ingredients:

Great quality coffee – The health benefits from butter coffee is increased if the coffee is of great quality. However, any coffee will do. Some recommend starting the Butter Coffee Weight Loss Protocol with whatever coffee brand or type (i.e., instant or brewed) is currently in use. Make sure that the taste of butter coffee is acceptable before venturing into a coffee upgrade.

Unsalted butter – Salt in coffee does not help improve the taste. It is a must to use the unsalted version of butter made from organically raised cows. That is, the source of the milk used in making the butter should come from free-range, grass-fed cows that were not treated with antibiotics or hormones. The most common butter brand certified to be made from milk of grass-fed cows is Kerry Gold. Never substitute unsalted butter in the recipe with salted ones or those made from non grass-fed cows. Most especially, never substitute with margarine. These will defeat the purpose of adding butter to coffee. These are unhealthy alternatives that will only add a huge chunk of unwanted calories and prevent weight loss.

MCT Oil – This can be found as a pure MCT product. Also, coconut oils contain a huge percentage of medium chain triglycerides that can be harnessed for the Butter Coffee Weight Loss Protocol. Pure MCT is more concentrated than coconut oils. Either can be used but MCT is found to be more potent and can help achieve weight loss faster.

- **Blender** – Water from coffee and oil never mix. A lot of people are put off by the oily layer floating on top of their morning joe. By placing the butter coffee and mixing them in a powerful blender, the oil can be better dispersed in the coffee, making it more palatable.

Procedure:

1. Start by brewing 1 cup (about 8 to 12 ounces) of coffee. Use filtered water and non-chlorinated. Add 2 ½ heaping tablespoon of freshly ground coffee.

2. Place the brewed coffee in a blender.

3. Add 1 to 2 tablespoon of MCT oil. Again, start small if not used to coconut oil or MCT. Best to start with 1 teaspoon and gradually

increase to the recommended 1-2 tablespoons.

4. Add 1 to 2 tablespoon of butter (unsalted and from grass-fed cows) or ghee.

5. Pulse in a blender for 20 to 30 seconds, until the mixture is frothy, resembling a frothy latte.

6. Pour into a cup and enjoy.

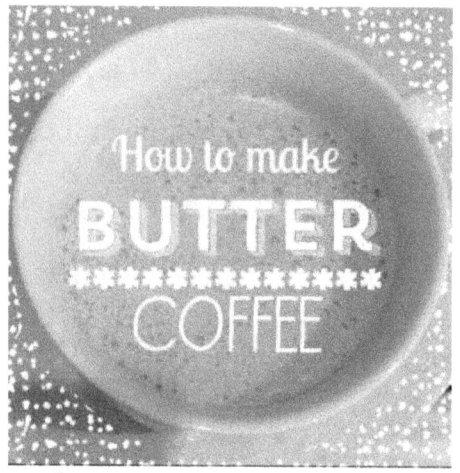

Image: http://www.workingmommagic.com/

Conclusion

Butter coffee is a fairly new beverage and a lot of debate is still ongoing regarding its benefits and effectiveness. The best way to find out is to judge it for yourself. Try this weight loss protocol today and find out for yourself if this really works or not. People react and reap benefits differently to certain weight loss regimens. The key to finding the one most fitted to one's needs is to try.

Get other people to join you in this journey. The support they can give can help you stick to the protocol and reap its rewards.

Thank you for purchasing this book and good luck in your journey towards weight loss, health and fitness.